Plant Powered Kitchen Cookbook

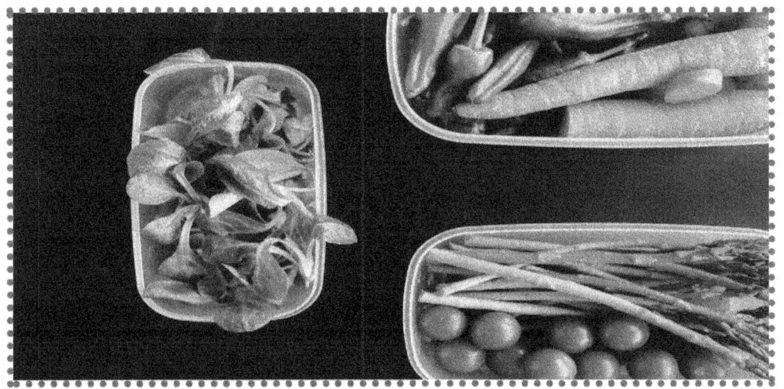

Quick and Easy Nutritious Recipes for a Healthy Lifestyle

Karla Mayer

TABLE OF CONTENT

INTRODUCTION

In a world where taste meets sustainability, where flavor and nourishment intertwine, a culinary journey awaits within the pages of the "Plant Powered Kitchen" cookbook. Venture into a realm where plants take center stage, elevating ordinary ingredients into extraordinary culinary creations.

Amidst the bustling cityscape, Karla, a passionate chef, found herself at a crossroads. Her heart yearned for a way to fuse her love for cooking with her deep-rooted concern for the environment. Inspired by the vibrant farmers' markets and the vivid colors of nature, she embarked on a quest to redefine the art of cooking.

The "Plant Powered Kitchen cookbook" unveils her remarkable odyssey. Each page whispers tales of innovative recipes that transcend boundaries, pushing the boundaries of conventional cuisine.

From the sizzle of savory grilled vegetables to the comforting embrace of hearty grain bowls, Karla's culinary expertise transforms plant-based ingredients into masterpieces that

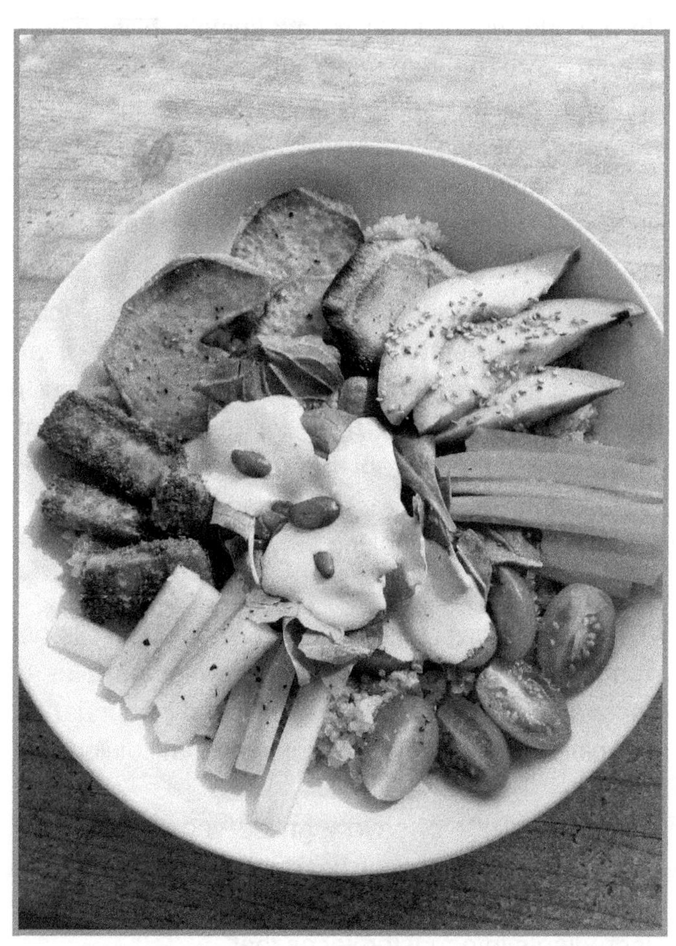

CHAPTER ONE

The Benefits of Plant-Based Eating

Plant-based eating offers numerous benefits for your health, the environment, and even animal welfare. Here's a detailed look at the advantages of adopting a plant-based diet:

1. Improved Health:
   - Heart Health: Plant-based diets are associated with lower risks of heart disease due to reduced intake of saturated fats and cholesterol. They can help lower blood pressure and cholesterol levels.
   - Weight Management: A plant-based diet can assist in weight loss and weight maintenance because it is typically lower in calories and

saturated fats, while being high in fiber, which promotes satiety.
  - Reduced Risk of Chronic Diseases: Studies show that plant-based diets are linked to a decreased risk of developing chronic conditions such as type 2 diabetes, certain cancers, and hypertension.

2. Nutrient-Rich Foods:
  - Plant-based diets emphasize whole, nutrient-dense foods like fruits, vegetables, legumes, nuts, and seeds, providing essential vitamins, minerals, and antioxidants crucial for overall health.

3. Environmental Benefits:
  - Reduced Greenhouse Gas Emissions: Plant-based diets have a lower carbon footprint compared to diets centered

around animal products.
Producing plant-based foods
typically generates fewer
greenhouse gases, helping
combat climate change.

- Conservation of Resources:
  Plant-based diets require less
  land, water, and energy
  compared to animal agriculture,
  contributing to the conservation
  of these vital resources.

4. Animal Welfare:

- Choosing plant-based foods
  helps reduce the demand for
  factory farming, thereby
  decreasing animal suffering. It
  aligns with ethical concerns for
  animal welfare.

5. Improved Digestion:

- Plant-based diets are often easier
  on the digestive system due to
  their high fiber content, promoting

regular bowel movements and a
healthy gut microbiome.

6. Reduced Risk of Foodborne Illnesses:
   - Plant-based diets are less
     susceptible to contamination with
     harmful bacteria and pathogens
     commonly associated with animal
     products.
7. Longevity: Some studies suggest that
   plant-based diets may contribute to a
   longer life span and a reduced risk of
   premature mortality.
8. Ethical and Moral Considerations:
   - Many individuals choose
     plant-based diets to align with
     their ethical beliefs and values,
     promoting a compassionate
     stance toward animals.
9. Cultural Diversity: Plant-based eating
   allows for a wide range of culinary
   diversity, with various cuisines offering
   delicious, meatless options, making it

accessible and enjoyable for people
from different cultural backgrounds.
10. Economic Benefits: Plant-based diets
can be cost-effective since grains,
legumes, and vegetables are often more
affordable than meat and dairy products.

Adopting a plant-based diet can have a
positive impact on your health, the
environment, and the well-being of animals. It's
a lifestyle choice that offers numerous benefits,
making it a compelling option for those looking
to lead a healthier and more sustainable life.

Essential Ingredients and Pantry Staples

Essential ingredients and pantry staples are the
foundation of a well-stocked kitchen. These items
provide the building blocks for countless recipes
and ensure you're prepared to cook a variety of
dishes at any time. Here are some essential
ingredients and pantry staples to keep on hand:

- Flour: All-purpose flour is versatile for baking and thickening sauces.
- Sugar: Granulated sugar, brown sugar, and powdered sugar are essential for baking and sweetening dishes.
- Salt: Regular table salt and kosher salt are used in seasoning and cooking.
- Pepper: Ground black pepper adds flavor to savory dishes.
- Olive Oil: A versatile cooking oil for sautéing, roasting, and salad dressings.
- Vegetable Oil: Ideal for frying and high-heat cooking.
- Vinegar: White vinegar, red wine vinegar, and balsamic vinegar are useful for dressings and marinades.
- Soy Sauce: Adds depth of flavor to Asian-inspired dishes.
- Pasta: Various types of pasta for quick and filling meals.
- Canned Tomatoes: Whole, diced, or crushed tomatoes are the base for many sauces and soups.

- Rice: Long-grain, short-grain, or basmati rice for a variety of dishes.
- Canned Beans: Black beans, kidney beans, and chickpeas are versatile and nutritious.
- Spices and Herbs: Common options include basil, oregano, garlic powder, and paprika.
- Onions and Garlic: Fresh and aromatic, they're essential for most savory dishes.
- Stock or Broth: Chicken, vegetable, or beef stock forms the base for soups and stews.
- Baking Powder and Baking Soda: Essential for leavening baked goods.
- Butter: Used in baking and for sautéing.
- Milk: Regular or non-dairy options for baking and cooking.
- Eggs: Versatile for baking, breakfast, and binding ingredients.
- Canned Tuna: A quick source of protein for salads and sandwiches.
- Honey and Maple Syrup: Natural sweeteners for both sweet and savory dishes.
- Nuts and Seeds: Almonds, walnuts, and sesame seeds add texture and flavor.

- Dried Pasta: Varieties like spaghetti, penne, and lasagna noodles are pantry staples.
- Cereal and Oats: Breakfast options that can also be used in baking.
- Cocoa Powder: For baking and making hot chocolate.
- Tea and Coffee: For a quick pick-me-up.
- Condiments: Ketchup, mustard, mayonnaise, and hot sauce for flavor enhancement.
- Canned Vegetables: Corn, peas, and green beans are convenient additions to meals.
- Canned Fruit: Pineapple, peaches, and mandarin oranges for desserts and snacks.
- Broth Cubes or Bouillon: A handy way to make broth if you don't have liquid stock.

Having these essential ingredients and pantry staples on hand allows you to whip up meals and snacks with ease, saving you time and ensuring you're ready for any culinary adventure. Regularly check and replenish these items to maintain a well-stocked pantry.

Tools and Equipment for Plant-Based Cooking

Here is a list of tools and equipment for plant-based cooking:

- High-Speed Blender: A powerful blender is essential for making smoothies, soups, sauces, and creamy plant-based desserts like cashew-based cheesecake.
- Food Processor: Ideal for chopping, slicing, and shredding vegetables, nuts, and fruits. It's useful for making veggie burgers, nut-based spreads, and energy bars.
- Mandoline Slicer: Makes uniform vegetable slices for salads, stir-fries, and vegetable chips.
- Chef's Knife: A good-quality chef's knife is crucial for precise chopping and slicing of vegetables and fruits.
- Cutting Boards: Invest in durable, eco-friendly cutting boards to prevent cross-contamination.
- Non-Stick Cookware: Pans with a non-stick surface are great for sautéing and stir-frying with less oil.

- Cast Iron Skillet: Perfect for searing, baking, and making one-pan plant-based dishes like tofu scrambles.
- Steamer Basket: Essential for cooking vegetables, grains, and dumplings while retaining nutrients.
- Spiralizer: Makes zucchini noodles (zoodles) and other veggie-based pasta alternatives.
- Nut Milk Bag: Essential for straining homemade nut milks and making plant-based cheeses.
- Silicone Baking Mats: Great for baking without parchment paper or greasing pans.
- Herb Mill or Mincer: For easily incorporating fresh herbs into your plant-based dishes.
- Citrus Juicer: Handy for adding fresh citrus juice to dressings, marinades, and beverages.

CHAPTER TWO

Breakfast and Brunch Delights

Energizing Smoothie Bowls

In a quaint kitchen nestled among the lush greenery of a peaceful neighborhood, Karla was starting her day with a burst of energy. The secret to her morning vitality? Energizing smoothie bowls.

Every morning, Karla would glide to her kitchen, her favorite music playing softly in the background. She would carefully select the freshest fruits from her garden – ripe bananas, plump strawberries, and juicy blueberries. These vibrant ingredients were the foundation of her daily ritual.As Karla sliced the bananas and washed the berries, she couldn't help but smile. She knew that within minutes, she would create a masterpiece that would not only nourish her body but also invigorate her spirit.With precision, she added the fruits to her blender, accompanied by a generous dollop of Greek yogurt and a splash of almond milk.

To enhance the nutritional value, she sprinkled in some chia seeds and a spoonful of honey. A quick whirl of the blender later, and her smoothie base was ready. Pouring the luscious mixture into a bowl, Karla began to decorate her creation. She meticulously placed sliced kiwi, a handful of crunchy granola, and a sprinkle of coconut flakes on top.

Each component added not only to the visual appeal but also to the burst of flavors and textures.As she took her first spoonful, a wave of refreshment and satisfaction swept over her. The sweet and creamy smoothie base danced on her taste buds, while the crunchy granola and chia seeds provided a satisfying contrast. The fresh fruit toppings exploded with natural sweetness, and the honey added a gentle touch of indulgence.

Karla savored each bite, her senses awakened and her body energized. With every spoonful, she felt ready to conquer the day ahead. Energized by the goodness of her homemade smoothie bowl, she tackled her tasks with enthusiasm, creativity, and a smile that seemed to shine a little brighter each morning.

And so, in her cozy kitchen surrounded by nature's beauty, Karla's daily ritual of preparing and enjoying energizing smoothie bowls became a cherished part of her life—a reminder that a wholesome and delicious breakfast can infuse every day with the vitality needed to embrace life's adventures.

Nutritious Overnight Oats Variation

Overnight oats have gained immense popularity for their convenience and health benefits. This versatile breakfast option offers a delicious way to kickstart your day with a nutritious punch. While the classic version is great, there are countless variations to explore, allowing you to customize your oats to suit your taste and dietary preferences.

Base Recipe

Start with rolled oats: These are the ideal oats for overnight preparation as they absorb liquid well.

Liquid: Use your choice of milk (dairy or plant-based) or yogurt for creaminess.

Sweetener: Honey, maple syrup, or agave nectar can add a touch of sweetness.

Mix-ins: Add fruits, nuts, seeds, or spices for flavor and texture.

Refrigerate: Combine all ingredients in a jar or container and refrigerate overnight.

Variations to Try

Fruity Delight: Mix in fresh berries, sliced banana, and a sprinkle of chia seeds. The natural sweetness of the fruits makes it a delightful choice.

Peanut Butter Bliss: Swirl in peanut butter for creaminess and top with sliced bananas and a drizzle of honey. It's like having a peanut butter sandwich in a jar.

Choco-Berry Indulgence: Add cocoa powder for a chocolatey twist and toss in some mixed berries for a burst of antioxidants.

Tropical Paradise: Incorporate diced pineapple, coconut flakes, and a dash of vanilla extract for a taste of the tropics.

Nutty Delight: Load up on chopped nuts (almonds, walnuts, or pecans), and mix in a dollop of almond or peanut butter for extra protein and crunch.

Pumpkin Spice Heaven: In the fall, try canned pumpkin puree, a sprinkle of pumpkin spice, and a touch of maple syrup for a cozy breakfast.

Green Goodness: Blend in spinach or kale for a vibrant green hue and a nutrient boost, then sweeten with banana and honey.

Nutritious overnight oats are a canvas for your culinary creativity. Whether you prefer fruity, nutty, chocolatey, or something entirely unique, you can craft a satisfying and healthful breakfast that suits your taste buds. With minimal effort the night before, you'll wake up to a delicious meal that keeps you energized throughout the morning. Experiment with these variations and discover your favorite way to enjoy this wholesome breakfast option.

Creative Avocado Toasts and Toppings

Avocado toast, a culinary canvas for the creative at heart, has taken the breakfast world by storm. Beyond its delicious simplicity lies a realm of endless possibilities for imaginative toppings that elevate this dish to a work of art.Start with a perfectly ripe avocado, its creamy green flesh begging to be spread across warm, toasted bread. The canvas is set, and now it's time to unleash your creativity.

Classic Elegance: Begin with a drizzle of extra virgin olive oil, a pinch of sea salt, and a twist of freshly ground black pepper. Top it off with a scattering of microgreens for a touch of color and earthy freshness.

Savory Sophistication: Transform your toast into a savory delight by adding thinly sliced smoked salmon and a dollop of herbed cream cheese. Cap it with finely chopped chives for a burst of flavor.

Mediterranean Magic: Transport your taste buds to the Mediterranean by layering on sun-dried tomatoes, crumbled feta cheese, and a sprinkle of za'atar seasoning. A drizzle of balsamic reduction adds the perfect finishing touch.

Spicy Fiesta: Spice things up with sliced jalapeños, a dash of smoked paprika, and a poached egg with a runny yolk. The creamy avocado tames the heat while the egg provides a luscious contrast.

Vegan Delight: For a vegan twist, mash avocado with lemon juice and spread it generously. Top with roasted cherry tomatoes, toasted pine nuts, and a swirl of tahini sauce for a rich and nutty flavor.

Tropical Paradise: Embrace the exotic by adding sliced mango, a sprinkle of chili flakes, and a handful of fresh cilantro leaves. The sweet and spicy combination is an explosion of taste.

Farmers' Market Bounty: Celebrate the season with fresh, locally sourced toppings. Think roasted beets, goat cheese crumbles, and a drizzle of honey for a symphony of flavors and colors.

Nutty Indulgence: Elevate your avocado toast by spreading almond or cashew butter on the bread before adding avocado slices. Sprinkle with crushed pistachios and a touch of honey for a delightful crunch and sweetness.

Remember, creativity knows no bounds when it comes to avocado toast. Whether you prefer sweet or savory, spicy or mild, there's a combination of toppings waiting to be discovered. So, grab that ripe avocado, toast your favorite bread, and let your culinary imagination soar. Each bite is a masterpiece of flavor and texture, a testament to the artistry of avocado toast.

CHAPTER THREE

Appetizers and Snacks

Fresh Vegetable Spring Rolls with Peanut Dipping

Fresh Vegetable Spring Rolls with Peanut Dipping Sauce are a delectable and healthy dish that combines the vibrant colors and flavors of fresh vegetables with the rich and creamy goodness of a homemade peanut sauce. Whether you're looking for a light appetizer, a refreshing snack, or a wholesome meal, these spring rolls are the perfect choice. In this article, we'll explore the ingredients, preparation, and the delightful journey of savoring these mouth watering spring rolls.

Ingredients for the Spring Rolls

Rice paper wrappers

Assorted fresh vegetables (lettuce, carrots, cucumber, bell peppers, bean sprouts, and fresh herbs like cilantro, mint, and basil)

Rice vermicelli noodles, cooked and cooled

Cooked shrimp or tofu (optional for added protein)

Rice vinegar for soaking rice paper wrappers (optional)

For the Peanut Dipping Sauce:

1/2 cup creamy peanut butter

2 tablespoons soy sauce

2 tablespoons rice vinegar

1 tablespoon honey or maple syrup

1 clove garlic, minced

1/2 teaspoon grated fresh ginger

A pinch of red pepper flakes (adjust to taste)

2-3 tablespoons warm water (for desired consistency)

Preparation: Prepare all your vegetables by thinly slicing them into long, thin strips. Keep them fresh and colorful for a visually appealing dish. Cook the rice vermicelli noodles according to package instructions, then rinse them with cold water and set aside. If using shrimp or tofu, cook and prepare them accordingly. Shrimp can be boiled and peeled, while tofu can be sliced into strips and pan-fried until lightly crispy.

To make the peanut dipping sauce, whisk together peanut butter, soy sauce, rice vinegar, honey, minced garlic, grated ginger, and red pepper flakes in a bowl. Add warm water gradually until you achieve your desired dipping consistency. Set aside.

Assembly: Fill a shallow dish with warm water. Take one rice paper wrapper and dip it into the water for a few seconds until it becomes pliable but not too soft. Lay it flat on a clean surface. Begin by placing a lettuce leaf on the lower third of the wrapper, leaving some space around the edges. Add a small handful of rice vermicelli noodles on top of the lettuce.Arrange your choice of vegetables, herbs, and protein (if using) on top of the noodles. Carefully fold the sides of the wrapper inward, then roll it up tightly from the bottom, making sure to enclose the filling completely. Repeat the process with the remaining ingredients.

Serving: Serve the fresh vegetable spring rolls with the homemade peanut dipping sauce on the side. They can be enjoyed as an appetizer, a light lunch, or a healthy snack. The combination of the crisp, fresh vegetables, the tender noodles, and the creamy peanut sauce creates a symphony of flavors and textures that's both satisfying and refreshing.

Fresh Vegetable Spring Rolls with Peanut Dipping Sauce are a delightful culinary adventure that offers a burst of freshness and flavor with every bite. Whether you're a seasoned cook or a beginner in the kitchen, these spring rolls are easy to prepare and will impress your friends and family. So, gather your ingredients, roll up your sleeves, and embark on a delicious journey into the world of fresh and wholesome Asian cuisine.

Roasted Chickpea Crunchies

Roasted Chickpea Crunchies are a delightful snack, marrying the earthy charm of chickpeas with the irresistible allure of a satisfying crunch. These golden nuggets undergo a transformation in the oven, becoming crisp and slightly toasted, releasing a symphony of flavors.

With each bite, you encounter a harmonious blend of nuttiness, warmth, and a hint of smokiness. The seasonings, whether savory or spicy, elevate the chickpeas to new heights, leaving your taste buds tantalized and craving more.But it's not just the taste; the texture of Roasted Chickpea Crunchies is equally enchanting.

Their initial firmness yields to a satisfying, airy crispness that provides a deeply satisfying eating experience.Whether you savor them as a stand alone snack or incorporate them into salads and trail mixes, Roasted Chickpea Crunchies are a testament to the culinary magic that can be achieved with a simple legume, transformed into a snack that is both wholesome and indulgent.

Savory Stuffed Mushrooms

Savory stuffed mushrooms are a delectable appetizer that combines the earthy richness of mushrooms with a flavorful filling, creating a harmonious burst of taste and texture in every bite. Whether served at a casual gathering or an elegant dinner party, these bite-sized wonders never fail to impress.

Ingredients

Fresh Mushrooms: Choose medium-sized white or cremini mushrooms, with firm caps.

Cream Cheese: Provides a creamy base for the filling.

Garlic: Minced garlic adds a subtle, aromatic kick.

Fresh Herbs: Parsley, thyme, or chives bring freshness and depth of flavor.

Breadcrumbs: Adds a crispy contrast to the tender mushrooms.

Parmesan Cheese: Grated parmesan lends a nutty, savory note.

Olive Oil: For drizzling and sautéing.

Instructions

Clean the mushrooms: Gently wipe the mushroom caps with a damp cloth to remove any dirt. Remove the stems and set them aside.

Prepare the filling

In a mixing bowl, combine cream cheese, minced garlic, finely chopped fresh herbs, breadcrumbs, and grated parmesan. Mix until well combined.

Stuff the mushrooms

Using a teaspoon, generously fill each mushroom cap with the cream cheese mixture, creating a small mound on top.

Bake

Place the stuffed mushrooms on a baking sheet, drizzle with olive oil, and bake in a preheated oven at 350°F (175°C) for about 15-20 minutes or until the mushrooms are tender and the filling is golden brown.

Serve and enjoy: Arrange the savory stuffed mushrooms on a serving platter, garnish with additional fresh herbs, if desired, and serve hot.

These delightful morsels are best enjoyed right out of the oven.Savory stuffed mushrooms are a versatile appetizer that can be customized to suit your taste. Experiment with different herb combinations, add a pinch of red pepper flakes for some heat, or incorporate finely chopped spinach or crab meat for an extra layer of flavor. Whether you're a seasoned cook or a novice in the kitchen, these savory stuffed mushrooms are sure to elevate your culinary repertoire and leave your guests craving for more.

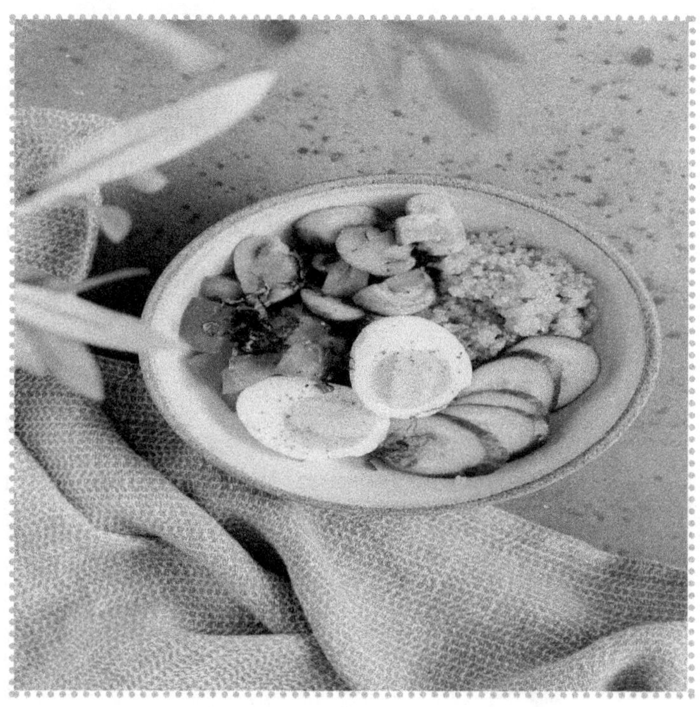

CHAPTER FOUR

Wholesome Soups and Salads

Creamy Butternut Squash Soup

Creamy butternut squash soup is a culinary masterpiece that transcends seasons, bringing warmth and comfort with every spoonful. Whether you're looking for a soul-soothing winter dish or a light and refreshing summer appetizer, this versatile soup has got you covered. Join us on a flavorful journey as we explore the essence of creamy butternut squash soup, from its humble roots to creative variations that will tantalize your taste buds.

The Art of Preparing Butternut Squash: The foundation of any great creamy butternut squash soup is, of course, the squash itself. Start by selecting a ripe, vibrant butternut squash, known for its sweet and nutty flavor. Roasting the squash brings out its natural sugars, intensifying the taste. Simply cut the squash in half, remove the seeds, brush with olive oil, sprinkle with salt and pepper, and roast until tender and caramelized.

The Essential Ingredients: Aside from the star ingredient, a few pantry staples are essential for creating that velvety texture and rich flavor. Onions, garlic, and a hint of nutmeg complement the sweetness of the butternut squash beautifully. For the creamy element, use heavy cream, coconut milk, or even Greek yogurt for a healthier twist. Don't forget to season with salt and pepper to taste.

Variations to Savor: Creamy butternut squash soup is a canvas for creativity. Here are some delightful variations to experiment with;

Apple Infusion: Add diced apples for a sweet and tart contrast.

Spicy Kick: A pinch of cayenne pepper or red pepper flakes adds an exciting heat.
Garnish Galore: Top your soup with roasted pumpkin seeds, croutons, or a drizzle of balsamic reduction for extra flair.

A Nutritional Powerhouse: Butternut squash is a nutritional powerhouse packed with vitamins, fiber, and antioxidants. It's an excellent source of vitamins A and C, which support your immune system, eye health, and skin. Plus, the fiber keeps you feeling full and satisfied.

Serving Suggestions: Creamy butternut squash soup can be served in various ways:
As a comforting bowl on its own.
Alongside a crisp salad for a balanced meal.
Paired with a grilled cheese sandwich for the ultimate cozy combo.
As an elegant appetizer in small cups at a dinner party

Seasonal Flexibility: One of the most remarkable aspects of creamy butternut squash soup is its adaptability. Serve it hot in the winter for a cozy evening in front of the fireplace, or serve it chilled in the summer as a refreshing, chilled gazpacho-style soup.

In every spoonful of creamy butternut squash soup, you'll find the perfect harmony of flavors and textures. It's a comforting classic that celebrates the bounty of autumn but can be enjoyed year-round. Whether you're a seasoned chef or a beginner in the kitchen, this soup is a must-try. So, grab a butternut squash, fire up your stove, and embark on a culinary journey that will warm your heart and soul. Creamy butternut squash soup is not just food; it's pure comfort in a bowl.

Fresh and Vibrant Kale Salad with Citrus Dressing

Elevate your salad game with this Fresh and Vibrant Kale Salad with Citrus Dressing. Packed with nutrient-rich kale, a medley of colorful vegetables, and a zesty citrus dressing, this salad is a burst of flavor and health in every bite. Whether you're looking for a light and refreshing side dish or a satisfying main course, this salad has got you covered. Let's dive into the recipe and discover how to create this delightful dish.

Ingredients for the Salad:

4 cups fresh kale leaves, stems removed and chopped

1 cup red cabbage, thinly sliced

1 large carrot, julienned

1 red bell pepper, thinly sliced

1/2 red onion, thinly sliced

1/4 cup dried cranberries

1/4 cup sliced almonds

1/4 cup crumbled feta cheese (optional)

For the Citrus Dressing:

1/4 cup freshly squeezed orange juice

2 tablespoons freshly squeezed lemon juice

2 tablespoons olive oil

1 tablespoon honey (or maple syrup for a vegan option)

1 teaspoon Dijon mustard

Salt and pepper to taste

Instructions in preparing the Kale:

Start by thoroughly washing the kale leaves and getting rid of the tough stems. Chop the kale into tiny-sized pieces and place them in a large salad bowl.

Massage the Kale: To make the kale more tender and flavorful, drizzle a little olive oil over the kale leaves and gently massage them for about 2-3 minutes. This helps to break down the fibers and reduce any bitterness.

Add Colorful Vegetables: Toss in the thinly sliced red cabbage, julienned carrot, red bell pepper, and red onion into the salad bowl with the kale. These vibrant veggies not only add color but also provide a variety of nutrients.

Sprinkle with Goodness: Scatter dried cranberries and sliced almonds over the salad for a delightful contrast of sweetness and crunchiness. If desired, sprinkle crumbled feta cheese on top for a creamy, tangy touch.

Make the Citrus Dressing: In a small bowl, whisk together the freshly squeezed orange juice, lemon juice, olive oil, honey (or maple syrup), Dijon mustard, salt, and pepper. Adjust the sweetness and tanginess to your liking.

Drizzle and Toss: Pour the citrus dressing over the salad and toss everything together until the ingredients are evenly coated with the vibrant dressing.

Let It Rest: Allow the salad to sit for about 10-15 minutes to let the flavors blend together and the kale soften further.

Serve and Enjoy: Plate your Fresh and Vibrant Kale Salad with Citrus Dressing and savor the burst of flavors. It's perfect as a light lunch, a side dish for dinner, or a healthy potluck contribution.

This Fresh and Vibrant Kale Salad with Citrus Dressing is a celebration of freshness, health, and taste. With the earthy flavor of kale, the crunch of colorful vegetables, and the zesty punch of the citrus dressing, this salad is a winner on every occasion. Whether you're a kale enthusiast or new to the world of leafy greens, this salad will undoubtedly become a favorite in your recipe collection. Give it a try today and you will be happy you did.

Creamy Roasted Tomato Soup with Cashew Cream

Creamy Roasted Tomato Soup with Cashew Cream is a delightful and nutritious twist on the classic tomato soup recipe. This dish combines the rich flavors of roasted tomatoes with the velvety texture of cashew cream, resulting in a satisfying and comforting meal. Here's a comprehensive overview of this delicious recipe:

Ingredients

Tomatoes: The star ingredient, ripe tomatoes are roasted to intensify their flavor. You can use a variety like Roma or vine-ripened tomatoes.

Cashews: Raw cashews are soaked and blended to create a creamy and dairy-free base for the soup.

Onions and Garlic: Sautéed onions and garlic add depth and aroma to the soup.

Vegetable Broth: Provides the liquid base and enhances the flavor. You can use homemade or store-bought vegetable broth.

Herbs and Spices: Common additions include fresh basil, thyme, salt, pepper, and a pinch of red pepper flakes for a subtle kick.

Olive Oil: Used for roasting the tomatoes and sautéing the onions and garlic.

Instructions

Roasting the Tomatoes: Preheat your oven to 400°F (200°C).Cut the tomatoes in half and place them on a baking sheet.Drizzle with olive oil, season with salt and pepper, and roast for about 30-40 minutes until they're soft and slightly caramelized. Soaking Cashews: Soak raw cashews in hot water for about 15-20 minutes until they become soft.

Sautéing Onions and Garlic:In a large pot, sauté finely chopped onions and minced garlic in olive oil until they turn translucent and aromatic.

Blending: Combine the roasted tomatoes, soaked cashews (drained), sautéed onions, and garlic in a blender. Add in fresh basil and other seasonings.

Blending and Simmering: Blend until you achieve a smooth, creamy consistency.Transfer the mixture back to the pot and add vegetable broth. Simmer the soup on low heat for about 10-15 minutes, allowing the flavors to meld.

Cashew Cream: While the soup simmers, prepare the cashew cream by blending soaked cashews with water until smooth and creamy. Pour the cashew cream into the soup, stirring gently to combine. Adjusting Seasonings:Taste and adjust the seasonings with salt, pepper, and a pinch of red pepper flakes if desired.

Serving: Ladle the creamy roasted tomato soup into bowls.Garnish with fresh basil leaves, a drizzle of olive oil, and a dollop of cashew cream. Serve hot with crusty bread or croutons.

Variations:You can customize this soup by adding roasted red peppers, carrots, or even a touch of balsamic vinegar for extra depth of flavor. For a creamier texture, you can use coconut milk or almond milk instead of cashew cream. Creamy Roasted Tomato Soup with Cashew Cream is a vegan and gluten-free option that's perfect for warming up on chilly days.

Its rich, velvety texture and the combination of roasted tomato flavors with the nutty creaminess of cashews make it a favorite comfort food for many. Enjoy this wholesome soup as a starter or a satisfying meal on its own.

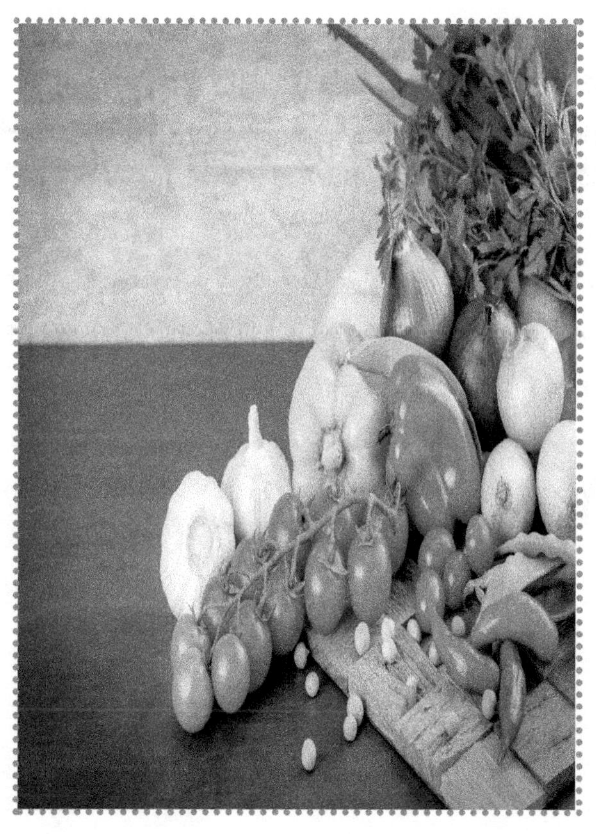

CHAPTER FIVE

Vibrant Main course

Zucchini Noodle Pesto Delight

Zucchini Noodles with Pesto and Cherry Tomatoes is a delightful and healthy dish that has gained popularity in recent years, particularly among those seeking low-carb or gluten-free alternatives to traditional pasta dishes. This recipe combines fresh, spiralized zucchini noodles with a vibrant homemade pesto sauce and sweet cherry tomatoes to create a flavorful and satisfying meal.

Ingredients:

1. Zucchini: Start with 3-4 medium-sized zucchinis. These will be spiralized into "noodles" using a spiralizer or julienne peeler.
2. Cherry Tomatoes: You'll need about 1 pint (2 cups) of cherry tomatoes. These

add a burst of sweetness and color to
the dish.

3. Pesto Sauce: You can either buy
   pre-made pesto sauce or make your
   own using fresh basil, garlic, pine nuts,
   Parmesan cheese, olive oil, and a pinch
   of salt. Blend these ingredients together
   until you achieve a smooth, vibrant
   green pesto sauce.

4. Olive Oil: For sautéing and enhancing
   the flavor of the dish.

5. Salt and Pepper: To season the noodles
   and tomatoes.

Instructions:

1. Prepare the Zucchini Noodles: Wash
   and trim the ends of the zucchinis.
   Using a spiralizer or julienne peeler, turn
   them into long, spaghetti-like noodles.
   Place the noodles in a colander, sprinkle
   with a little salt, and let them sit for
   about 10-15 minutes. This helps draw

out excess moisture. After that, pat them dry with paper towels.

2. Cook the Cherry Tomatoes: In a large skillet, heat some olive oil over medium heat. Add the cherry tomatoes and cook them until they start to blister and burst, releasing their juices. This usually takes about 5-7 minutes. Season to taste with salt and pepper.

3. Sauté the Zucchini Noodles: In another skillet, heat some more olive oil over medium-high heat. Add the zucchini noodles and stir-fry them for 2-3 minutes until they are tender but not overly soft, so as to retain a level of crunchiness.

4. Combine Everything: Add the sautéed zucchini noodles to the skillet with the cherry tomatoes. Pour in your homemade or store-bought pesto sauce and toss everything together until the noodles and tomatoes are coated evenly with the pesto.

5. Serve: Plate the zucchini noodles with pesto and cherry tomatoes, and if desired, garnish with fresh basil leaves and extra grated Parmesan cheese. You can also sprinkle some pine nuts for extra texture and flavor.

This dish is not only visually appealing but also a nutritious alternative to traditional pasta. The zucchini noodles provide a light and refreshing base, while the pesto sauce and cherry tomatoes offer a burst of flavor. It's a perfect option for those looking to incorporate more vegetables into their diet or simply enjoy a delicious, gluten-free meal. Feel free to customize it with additional ingredients like grilled chicken or shrimp for added protein or a sprinkle of red pepper flakes for some heat.

Spicy Chickpea Curry with Fragrant Basmati Rice

Spicy Chickpea Curry with Fragrant Basmati Rice is a culinary adventure that mixes the comfort of rice with the warmth of spices. This vegetarian dish is a beautiful combination of flavors and fragrances that will take your taste senses to India's bustling streets. Join us as we uncover the secrets to making this delectable feast.

Ingredients:
For the Spicy Chickpea Curry, prepare the following:

2 cups chickpeas cooked (canned or soaked and boiling)

2 tbsp of vegetable oil

1 large onion, finely chopped 3 garlic cloves, minced 1 inch piece ginger, grated

2 chopped tomatoes

1 cup canned coconut milk

2 tablespoons cumin and 2 teaspoons coriander

1 teaspoon turmeric powder

1/2 teaspoon red chili powder (modify according to taste)

Season with salt to taste

Garnish with fresh cilantro leaves

To prepare the Fragrant Basmati Rice:

1 casserole Basmati rice

2 c. water

2-3 cardamom pods, green

1 stick cinnamon

4 to 5 cloves

one bay leaf

Season with salt to taste

Instructions:

Rinse the Basmati rice completely and soak it for 30 minutes in water. The rice should be drained.

In a large saucepan over medium heat, heat the vegetable oil. Sauté the chopped onions until they turn translucent.

Cook for a few minutes more, until the minced garlic and grated ginger are aromatic.

Mix in the ground cumin, coriander, turmeric, and red chili powder. Allow the spices to roast for a minute to release their flavors.

Cook until the tomatoes are softened

Bring the mixture to a gentle simmer after adding the coconut milk.

Season with salt and pepper to taste. enable the curry to simmer for 10-15 minutes to enable the flavors to blend and the chickpeas to absorb the delectable sauce.

Prepare the aromatic Basmati rice while the curry simmers. Add the drained rice, water, green cardamom pods, cinnamon stick, cloves, bay leaf, and a bit of salt to a separate pot.

Bring to a boil, then lower to a low heat, cover, and leave to simmer until the rice is tender and the water has been absorbed.

When the rice and chickpea curry are done, combine them on a plate. For a pop of color and taste, garnish with fresh cilantro leaves.

Spicy Chickpea Curry with Fragrant Basmati Rice is a delectable and gratifying recipe that combines aromatic Indian spices with the subtle elegance of Basmati rice. Whether you're a spice connoisseur or just looking for a hearty vegetarian supper, this recipe will satisfy your taste buds and leave you wanting more. With each bite, enjoy the mix of flavors and the fragrant journey it takes you on.

Creamy Cashew Alfredo Pasta

Cashew Alfredo Pasta is a dairy-free and vegan alternative to traditional Alfredo sauce. It's made by blending soaked cashews with ingredients like garlic, nutritional yeast, lemon juice, and vegetable broth to create a rich and creamy sauce. Here's a precise recipe:

Ingredients:

- 1 cup raw cashews, soaked for 30 minutes in boiling water

- 2 cloves garlic, minced
- 1/4 cup nutritional yeast
- 2 tablespoons lemon juice
- 1 cup vegetable broth
- Salt and pepper to taste
- 12 ounces fettuccine or your preferred pasta
- Fresh parsley for garnish (optional)

Instructions:

1. Cook the pasta according to the package directions until it is al dente. Set aside after draining..
2. In a high-speed blender, combine the soaked cashews, minced garlic, nutritional yeast, lemon juice, vegetable broth, salt, and pepper. Blend until the mixture is smooth and creamy, adding more broth if needed for desired consistency.

3. In a saucepan over medium heat, pour the cashew sauce and warm it, stirring frequently. Be careful not to let it boil. Taste and adjust seasoning as necessary.

4. Once the sauce is heated through, pour it over the cooked pasta and toss to coat evenly.

5. Serve the Creamy Cashew Alfredo Pasta hot, garnished if desired with fresh parsley.

This plant-based Alfredo pasta is rich, creamy, and satisfying without the use of dairy. It's a great option for those with dietary restrictions or anyone looking for a delicious and healthier pasta sauce alternative.

CHAPTER SIX

Indulgent Desserts

Rich Chocolate Avocado Mousse

Rich Chocolate Avocado Mousse is a delectable dessert that combines the creamy goodness of ripe avocados with the indulgent richness of dark chocolate. This innovative and healthier take on traditional mousse is not only a treat for your taste buds but also a guilt-free delight.

Ingredients:

- 2 ripe avocados
- 1/4 cup cocoa powder (unsweetened)
- 1/4 cup maple syrup or honey (according to taste)

- 1/4 cup almond milk (or other milk of choice)
- 1 teaspoon vanilla extract
- A pinch of salt
- 3-4 tablespoons dark chocolate chips or shavings for garnish (optional)
- Garnish with fresh berries or chopped nuts (optional).

Instructions:

1. Prepare the Avocados: Cut the avocados in half, remove the pits, and scoop the flesh into a blender or food processor.
2. Blend: Add the cocoa powder, maple syrup (or honey), almond milk, vanilla extract, and a pinch of salt to the blender with the avocados. Blend until smooth and creamy.. You may need to scrape down the sides of the blender or

food processor a few times to ensure everything is well combined.

3. Taste and Adjust: Taste the mousse and adjust the sweetness to your liking by adding more maple syrup or honey if needed. Blend again to combine.

4. Chill: Transfer the chocolate avocado mixture into individual serving glasses or bowls. Refrigerate for at least 30 minutes to let it to cold and set.

5. Garnish: Before serving, you can garnish each portion with dark chocolate chips or shavings for an extra burst of chocolate flavor and some fresh berries or chopped nuts for added texture and freshness.

6. Enjoy: Serve your Rich Chocolate Avocado Mousse chilled and savor the velvety texture and decadent chocolate taste with the added benefit of healthy fats from the avocados.

This dessert not only satisfies your sweet tooth but also provides the nutritional benefits of avocados, which are packed with vitamins, minerals, and healthy fats. It's a perfect treat for anyone looking for a healthier dessert option without compromising on flavor and indulgence.

Moist and Fudgy Vegan Brownies

Vegan brownies have come a long way from being considered a compromise in taste and texture. With the right ingredients and techniques, you can create brownies that are every bit as moist and fudgy as their non-vegan counterparts. In this article, we'll explore how to make the most delicious, moist and fudgy vegan brownies that will satisfy your chocolate cravings and leave you wanting more.

Ingredients:

1. 1 cup all-purpose flour
2. 1 cup granulated sugar
3. 1/2 cup unsweetened cocoa powder
4. 1/2 tsp baking powder
5. 1/2 tsp salt
6. 1/2 cup unsweetened applesauce
7. 1/4 vegetable oil
8. 1/4 cup almond milk (or plant-based milk of choice)
9. 1 tablespoon vanilla extract
10. 1/2 cup vegan chocolate chips

Instructions:

1. Preheat your oven to 350°F (175°C) and line an 8x8-inch (20x20 cm) baking pan with parchment paper, leaving some overhang for easy removal.

2. Whisk together the flour, sugar, cocoa powder, baking powder, and salt in a large mixing basin until well blended

3. Add the unsweetened applesauce, vegetable oil, almond milk, and vanilla extract to the dry ingredients. Mix until you have a smooth and thick batter.

4. If you want to take your vegan brownies to the next level, fold in the vegan chocolate chips. This will increase the richness and decadence.

5. Spread the brownie batter evenly in the prepared baking sheet.

6. Bake in the preheated oven for 25-30 minutes or until a toothpick inserted into the center comes out with a few moist crumbs. Be careful not to overbake; you want these brownies to be moist and fudgy.

7. Remove the brownies from the oven and let them cool for about 10 minutes in the pan. Then, use the parchment

paper over-hang to lift them out of the pan and onto a wire rack to cool completely.

8. Once cooled, cut the brownies into squares and indulge in their moist, fudgy goodness.

These moist and fudgy vegan brownies are a testament to how satisfying and delicious vegan desserts can be. With simple substitutions like applesauce and almond milk, you can create a treat that's just as enjoyable as traditional brownies, all while being cruelty-free. Whether you're a vegan or just looking to reduce your dairy intake, give this recipe a try and savor the chocolatey goodness in every bite.

Diary-Free Banana Nice Cream with Toppings

Craving a sweet and creamy treat but want to skip the dairy? Look no further than this delectable Diary-free Banana Nice Cream with Toppings. This guilt-free dessert is not only easy to make but also incredibly delicious, making it the perfect choice for anyone with a sweet tooth and dietary preferences. Let's dive into the world of creamy banana goodness and explore the endless topping possibilities that will elevate your dessert game.

Ingredients:

- 4 ripe bananas
- 2 tablespoons of almond or coconut milk (or your preferred dairy-free alternative)
- 1 teaspoon of pure vanilla extract
- A pinch of salt
- Toppings of your choice (see suggestions below)

Instructions:

1. Peel and Slice: Start by peeling the ripe bananas and slicing them into coins. Pro tip: You can freeze the banana slices in advance for an even creamier texture.
2. Freeze: Place the banana slices in a single layer on a baking sheet and freeze for at least 2 hours or until they are completely frozen. This step is crucial for achieving the creamy ice cream-like consistency.
3. Blend: Once the banana slices are frozen, transfer them to a high-powered blender or food processor. Add the dairy-free milk, pure vanilla extract, and a pinch of salt. Blend until smooth and creamy, scraping down the sides as necessary
4. Serve: Scoop the luscious banana nice cream into bowls or cones.

Topping Ideas:

1. Fresh Berries: Top your banana nice cream with a colorful assortment of fresh berries

like strawberries, blueberries, and raspberries. The natural sweetness and vibrant colors will complement the creamy banana base.

2. Crunchy Nuts: Add some texture and healthy fats with a sprinkle of chopped nuts such as almonds, walnuts, or pecans. Toasted nuts can add an extra dimension of flavor.

3. Chocolate Drizzle: For a touch of indulgence, drizzle dairy-free dark chocolate or vegan chocolate sauce over your nice cream. It's a heavenly combination with the banana's natural sweetness.

4. Nut Butter Swirl: Swirl in a generous dollop of your favorite nut butter, whether it's almond, peanut, or cashew butter. The rich, nutty flavor pairs wonderfully with the creamy banana base.

5. Coconut Shavings: Sprinkle some toasted coconut flakes on top for a tropical twist. It adds a delightful crunch and a hint of exotic flavor.

Diary-free Banana Nice Cream with Toppings is the perfect dessert for those seeking a healthier, plant-based alternative to traditional ice cream. It's not only dairy-free but also bursting with natural banana sweetness and endless topping possibilities. Whether you're enjoying it on a hot summer day or as a guilt-free late-night treat, this creamy delight is sure to satisfy your cravings while keeping your dietary choices in check. So, gather your favorite toppings and whip up a batch of this heavenly treat today.

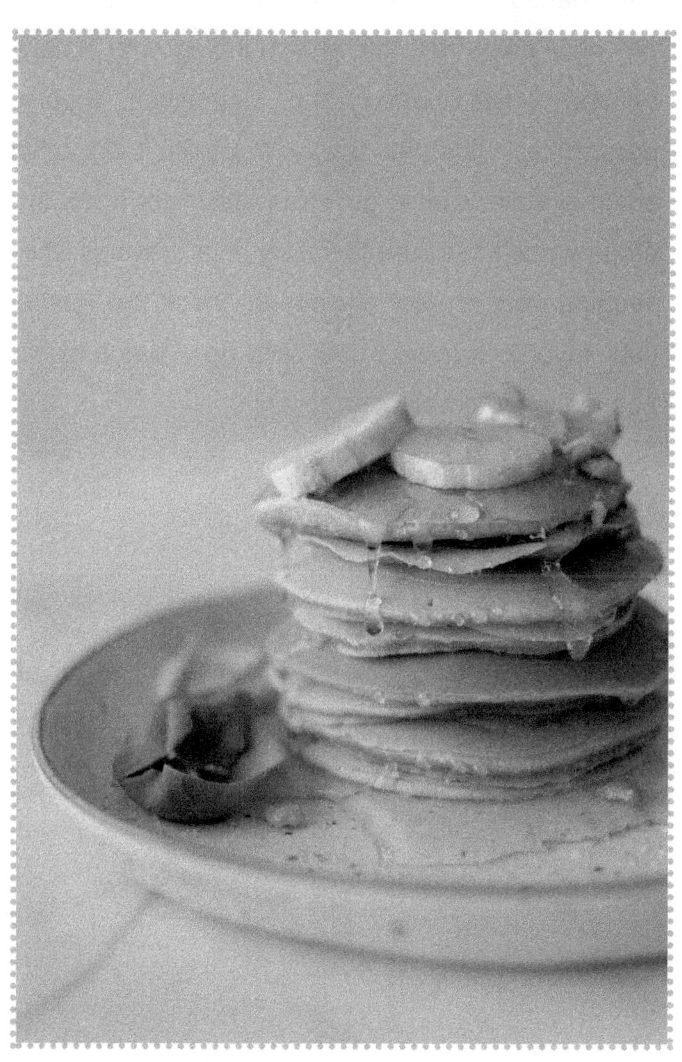

CHAPTER SEVEN

Drinks and Refreshments

Refreshing Watermelon and Mint Cooler

As the sun beats down during scorching summer days, there's nothing quite like sipping on a cool, revitalizing drink to beat the heat. One such delightful and hydrating beverage is the Watermelon and Mint Cooler. This invigorating concoction combines the sweet, juicy essence of watermelon with the refreshing burst of mint, creating the perfect summer refreshment.

Ingredients:

To make this revitalizing cooler, you'll need the following ingredients:

- 4 cups fresh watermelon chunks (seeded)

- 1/2 cup of fresh mint leaves
- 2 tablespoons of honey or agave nectar (adjust to taste)
- 1 tablespoon of fresh lime juice (optional)
- Ice cubes for serving
- Mint sprigs and watermelon wedges for garnish

Instructions:

Chill the Ingredients:

Start by ensuring that your watermelon chunks are chilled. You can also refrigerate your serving glasses beforehand for an extra refreshing experience.

Blend Watermelon and Mint:
In a blender, combine the chilled watermelon chunks and fresh mint leaves. Blend until you achieve a smooth and vibrant pink mixture.

Sweeten to Taste:

Depending on the sweetness of your watermelon, add honey or agave nectar to the blender. Start with 2 tablespoons and adjust according to your preference. For a zesty twist, you can also add a tablespoon of fresh lime juice.

Strain (Optional):

If you prefer a smoother texture without mint bits, strain the mixture through a fine-mesh sieve into a large pitcher.

Serve with Ice:

Fill your chilled glasses with ice cubes and pour the watermelon-mint mixture over the ice.

Garnish:

For an elegant touch, garnish your Watermelon and Mint Cooler with a sprig of fresh mint and a small watermelon wedge on the rim of each glass.

Enjoy:

Sip slowly and relish the sweet, hydrating, and revitalizing flavors of this summer cooler. It's the perfect remedy for hot, sunny days.

Health Benefits:

Apart from its delicious taste, this Watermelon and Mint Cooler offers several health benefits:

- Hydration: Watermelon is rich in water content, keeping you hydrated.
- Nutrient-Rich: Watermelon is a good source of vitamins A and C, while mint provides a refreshing burst of flavor.
- Digestive Aid: Mint can help soothe digestive discomfort.
- Low in Calories: It's a guilt-free beverage that's perfect for those watching their calorie intake.

The Watermelon and Mint Cooler is not just a thirst-quenching drink; it's a celebration of summer's bounty. With its delightful blend of watermelon's sweetness and mint's freshness, this cooler is a must-try for anyone looking to beat the heat and stay refreshed. So, grab your ingredients, blend up a batch, and let the cool, revitalizing flavors transport you to a summer paradise. Cheers to remaining cool and rejuvenated throughout the summer.

Creamy and Nutritious Green Smoothie

A creamy and nutritious green smoothie is a delightful way to kickstart your day with a burst of energy and essential nutrients. Packed with vitamins, minerals, fiber, and healthy fats, this vibrant green concoction not only tastes delicious but also offers a multitude of health benefits. In this article, we will explore the ingredients, preparation, and the nutritional advantages of this green smoothie.

Ingredients:

1. Leafy Greens: Begin with a generous handful of nutrient-rich leafy greens such as spinach, kale, or Swiss chard. These greens are low in calories but high in vitamins A, C, and K, as well as minerals like iron and calcium.

2. Creamy Base: To achieve that velvety texture, add a creamy base like Greek yogurt, almond milk, or avocado. These ingredients provide protein, healthy fats, and a satisfying thickness to the smoothie.

3. Fresh Fruits: Incorporate fruits for natural sweetness and additional vitamins. Common choices include bananas, apples, or pineapple. They contribute vitamins, antioxidants, and fiber.

4. Protein: To make your smoothie more filling, consider adding a scoop of

protein powder, nut butter, or hemp
seeds. This boosts protein content,
promoting satiety and muscle recovery.

5. Healthy Fats: A source of healthy fats
    like chia seeds, flaxseeds, or almond
    butter can enhance the creaminess
    while providing omega-3 fatty acids,
    promoting heart and brain health.

6. Flavor Enhancers: Enhance the taste
    with a touch of honey, vanilla extract, or
    a pinch of cinnamon. These ingredients
    add a subtle sweetness and aroma to
    your smoothie.

Preparation:

1. Start by washing and preparing your
    leafy greens, fruits, and any additional
    ingredients.
2. Place the leafy greens in the blender
    first, followed by the creamy base, fruits,
    protein, and healthy fats.

3. Add flavor enhancers and any optional ingredients.

4. Blend until smooth and creamy. If necessary, adjust the consistency by adding more liquid or ice cubes.

5. Taste and adjust sweetness or flavor to your preference.

Nutritional Benefits:

- High in Vitamins and Minerals: The leafy greens and fruits provide an abundance of essential vitamins and minerals, including vitamin C, potassium, and folate.
- Fiber-Rich: This smoothie is packed with dietary fiber, which aids digestion and keeps you feeling full.
- Protein-Packed: Protein from the creamy base and additional protein sources helps maintain muscle mass and promotes overall satiety.

- Healthy Fats: The inclusion of healthy fats supports heart health and can help regulate cholesterol levels.
- Antioxidant-Rich: Fruits and leafy greens are rich in antioxidants, which combat oxidative stress and promote overall well-being.

A creamy and nutritious green smoothie is a versatile and wholesome addition to your daily routine. Whether you're looking to boost your energy levels, increase your nutrient intake, or simply savor a delicious treat, this green smoothie offers it all. Experiment with different combinations of ingredients to find your perfect blend and enjoy the countless health benefits it provides.

Energizing Matcha Latte with Plant-Based Milk

Discover a revitalizing way to start your day with an Energizing Matcha Latte made with plant-based milk. This vibrant green elixir combines the rich, earthy flavors of matcha green tea with the creaminess of plant-based milk, creating a harmonious blend that not only tantalizes your taste buds but also nourishes your body.

Matcha, a finely ground green tea powder, is renowned for its numerous health benefits. It's packed with antioxidants, vitamins, and minerals, providing a natural energy boost without the jitters of caffeine. When combined with plant-based milk, such as almond, soy, or oat milk, this latte becomes a dairy-free, vegan-friendly delight that suits various dietary preferences.

The process is simple: whisk a teaspoon of matcha powder into a small amount of hot water to create a smooth paste. Then, gently heat your plant-based milk of choice, making sure not to bring it to a boil. Pour the warm milk into the matcha paste, sweeten to your liking with honey or maple syrup, and stir. The result is a velvety, green concoction that feels like a warm hug for your senses.

Not only does this Energizing Matcha Latte provide a gentle caffeine kick, but it also promotes mental clarity and a sense of calm. Its vibrant green color reflects its vitality, offering a visual treat as well. Sip, savor, and let this delightful beverage set a positive tone for your day, leaving you feeling refreshed, focused, and ready to conquer whatever lies ahead.

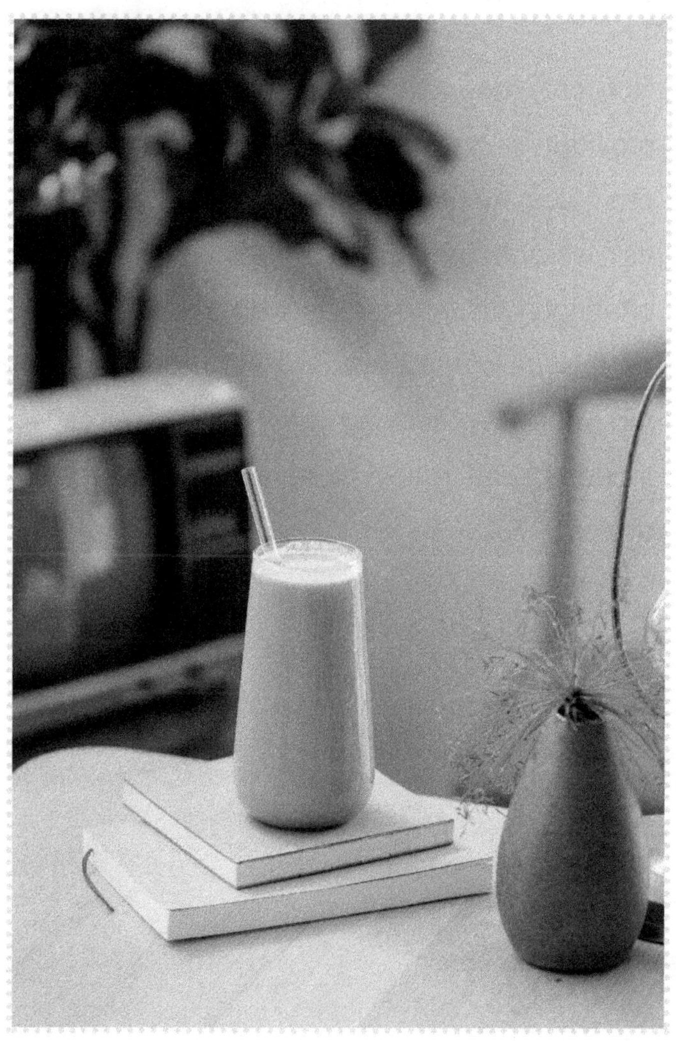

CHAPTER EIGHT

Tips for Vegan Success

How to Substitute Animal Products in Recipes

Substituting animal products in recipes is a wonderful way to embrace a more plant-based or vegan lifestyle while still enjoying delicious meals. Here are some tips and ideas on how to make these substitutions seamlessly:

1. Plant-Based Milks: Replace cow's milk with plant-based alternatives like almond, soy, oat, or coconut milk. These options work well in most recipes, including baking, cooking, and beverages.
2. Egg Replacements:
   - Flax or Chia Eggs: Mix 1 tablespoon of ground flaxseeds or chia seeds with 3 tablespoons

of water to replace one egg in recipes.

- Applesauce or Mashed Banana: Use 1/4 cup of unsweetened applesauce or mashed banana for each egg in baking recipes.
- Silken Tofu: Blend 1/4 cup of silken tofu until smooth to replace one egg in recipes like quiches and custards.

3. Plant-Based Butter: Swap dairy butter for vegan alternatives made from coconut, avocado, or almond. These work well in both baking and cooking.

4. Plant-Based Yogurt: Substitute dairy yogurt with soy, almond, or coconut yogurt in recipes, such as smoothies, dips, and marinades.

5. Cheese Alternatives: There's a wide variety of vegan cheeses available, or you can make your own from cashews or almonds. They work wonderfully in

dishes like lasagna, pizza, or as a topping for nachos.

6. Meat Substitutes:
    ○ Tofu: Press and marinate tofu for a versatile meat replacement in stir-fries, sandwiches, and salads.
    ○ Tempeh: A fermented soybean product with a nutty flavor, great for grilling, stir-frying, or crumbling into dishes.
    ○ Seitan: A high-protein wheat gluten product that mimics the texture of meat, suitable for recipes like stir-fries and sandwiches.
    ○ Mushrooms: Portobello mushrooms can be grilled or roasted for a meaty texture in burgers and sandwiches.
7. Nutritional Yeast: This provides a cheesy flavor and is perfect for

sprinkling on pasta, popcorn, or in vegan sauces.

8. Aquafaba: The liquid from canned chickpeas can be whipped into a foam to replace egg whites in recipes like meringues and macarons.

9. Spices and Herbs: Experiment with a variety of herbs and spices to enhance the flavors of your plant-based dishes. Smoked paprika, nutritional yeast, and liquid smoke can add depth to dishes.

10. Experiment and Adapt: Don't be afraid to experiment and adapt your favorite recipes. It may take a few tries to get the perfect substitution, but the journey can be delicious and rewarding.

Remember that the key to successful animal product substitutions is to be open to new flavors and textures. With creativity and practice, you can enjoy the benefits of plant-based cooking without sacrificing taste or variety in your meals. Happy cook.

Meal Planning for Success

Meal planning is a key strategy for achieving success in maintaining a healthy diet and achieving your nutritional goals. Whether you're aiming to lose weight, gain muscle, or simply eat better, effective meal planning can be a game-changer. In this guide, we will explore the importance of meal planning and provide practical tips to help you prepare for success in your nutrition journey.

Understand Your Goals:

1. Before diving into meal planning, it's essential to have clear nutritional goals. Are you trying to lose weight, build muscle, or simply eat a balanced diet? Knowing your objectives will guide your meal planning decisions.

Create a Weekly Menu:

2. Plan your meals for the week ahead. Designate specific days for breakfast, lunch, dinner, and snacks. Having a menu helps you make healthier choices and reduces the temptation of ordering takeout.

Balanced Nutrition:

3. Ensure your meals include a balance of macronutrients – carbohydrates, proteins, and fats. Include plenty of vegetables and fruits for vitamins and minerals. Adjust portion sizes based on your calorie needs.

Grocery Shopping:

4. Make a shopping list based on your
    weekly menu. Stick to your shopping list
    to avoid impulse purchases.. Shopping
    with a full stomach can also help you
    make better choices.

Prep in Advance:

5. Save time during the week by prepping
    ingredients in advance. Chop
    vegetables, cook grains, and marinate
    proteins. Having prepped ingredients on
    hand makes meal assembly a breeze.

Portion Control:

6. Invest in portion control tools like
    measuring cups and a food scale.
    Proper portioning can help you avoid

overeating and stay on track with your dietary goals.

Healthy Snacks:

7. Stock your kitchen with healthy snacks like nuts, yogurt, or fruit. This prevents reaching for unhealthy options when you're hungry between meals.

Meal Diversity:

8. Don't fall into a rut by eating the same meals every day. Experiment with different recipes and cuisines to keep your meals exciting and enjoyable.

Stay Hydrated:

9. Remember to stay hydrated throughout
    the day. Sometimes, thirst is mistaken
    for hunger.

Monitor Progress:

10. Track your meals and their impact on
    your goals. Use a journal or a nutrition
    app to record what you eat and how it
    makes you feel. Adjust your meal plan
    as needed.

Flexibility:

11. Life can be unpredictable. Be flexible
    with your meal plan and don't stress if
    you occasionally deviate from it. The

key is to maintain a long-term,
sustainable approach.

Meal planning and preparation are essential tools for success in achieving your nutritional goals. By understanding your objectives, creating balanced menus, and staying organized, you can set yourself up for success on your journey towards a healthier, happier you. Remember, consistency is key, and small, sustainable changes can lead to significant improvements in your overall well-being.

Navigating Social Situations and Eating Out

Eating out in social situations can be enjoyable and stress-free with a few key strategies:

1. Choose the Right Restaurant: Pick a restaurant with a diverse menu that accommodates various dietary

preferences. Research the menu online beforehand if possible.

2. Plan Ahead: If you have dietary restrictions or allergies, inform your host or the restaurant staff in advance. They can often provide suitable options or make adjustments.

3. Mindful Ordering: When ordering, consider healthier choices like salads, lean proteins, or grilled options. Portion control is vital; you can ask for half-sized portions or share dishes with a friend.

4. Etiquette Matters: Good table manners go a long way in social situations. Close your mouth when chewing, use utensils properly, and speak politely.

5. Alcohol Moderation: If alcohol is involved, drink responsibly. It's okay to decline if you prefer not to consume alcohol.

6. Engage Socially: Focus on the company and conversation rather than just the

food. This makes the experience more enjoyable and less about dietary concerns.

7. Be Flexible: Sometimes, you may not find the perfect option. In such cases, be flexible and make the best choice available without stressing over it.

8. Gratitude: Always express gratitude to your host or the restaurant staff. It's a simple way to show appreciation for the experience.

By following these tips, you can navigate social situations and dining out with confidence, ensuring a pleasant experience for both you and your companions.

CHAPTER NINE

Embracing the Plant Powered Lifestyle

Vegan Cooking: Joy & Flavor

Vegan cooking has come a long way from being seen as a niche dietary choice. Today, it has gained widespread recognition for its delicious flavors, health benefits, and positive impact on the environment. This celebration of vegan cooking is not just about dietary restrictions; it's a culinary journey filled with joy, creativity, and an explosion of flavors.

The Evolution of Vegan Cuisine:

1. Vegan cooking has evolved significantly over the years. It's no longer about simply replacing animal products with plant-based alternatives. Chefs and

home cooks alike have embraced the challenge of creating innovative and mouthwatering dishes that rival traditional favorites.

The Joy of Ingredients:

2. Vegan cooking celebrates the beauty and variety of plant-based ingredients. From colorful vegetables to exotic grains and legumes, the array of choices is endless. This diversity invites experimentation and sparks joy in the kitchen.

Flavor Explosion:

3. Contrary to misconceptions, vegan food is far from bland. With the right spices, herbs, and cooking techniques, vegan dishes burst with flavor. Savory curries,

zesty salads, and decadent desserts are just a few examples of the taste sensations waiting to be explored.

Health Benefits:

4. One of the joys of vegan cooking is its inherent health benefits. A well-balanced vegan diet can reduce the risk of chronic diseases, promote weight loss, and boost overall vitality. Knowing that every bite contributes to your well-being adds to the satisfaction of cooking vegan.

Environmental Impact:

5. Celebrating vegan cooking goes beyond the plate. It acknowledges the positive impact on our planet. By choosing plant-based ingredients over animal

products, we reduce greenhouse gas emissions, conserve water resources, and protect ecosystems.

Creativity in the Kitchen:

6. Vegan cooking encourages creativity and culinary exploration. It challenges cooks to think outside the box, experiment with new flavors, and invent innovative dishes. This element of creativity adds an exciting dimension to vegan cooking.

Inclusivity and Compassion:

7. Vegan cooking celebrates inclusivity and compassion. It accommodates various dietary preferences and respects the welfare of animals. Sharing vegan

meals with others fosters a sense of community and understanding

Celebrating the joy and flavor of vegan cooking is an ode to the vibrant world of plant-based cuisine. It's about savoring diverse ingredients, exploring bold flavors, and contributing to a healthier planet. Whether you're a seasoned vegan chef or just starting your journey, the joy of vegan cooking is an experience worth savoring, one delicious dish at a time.

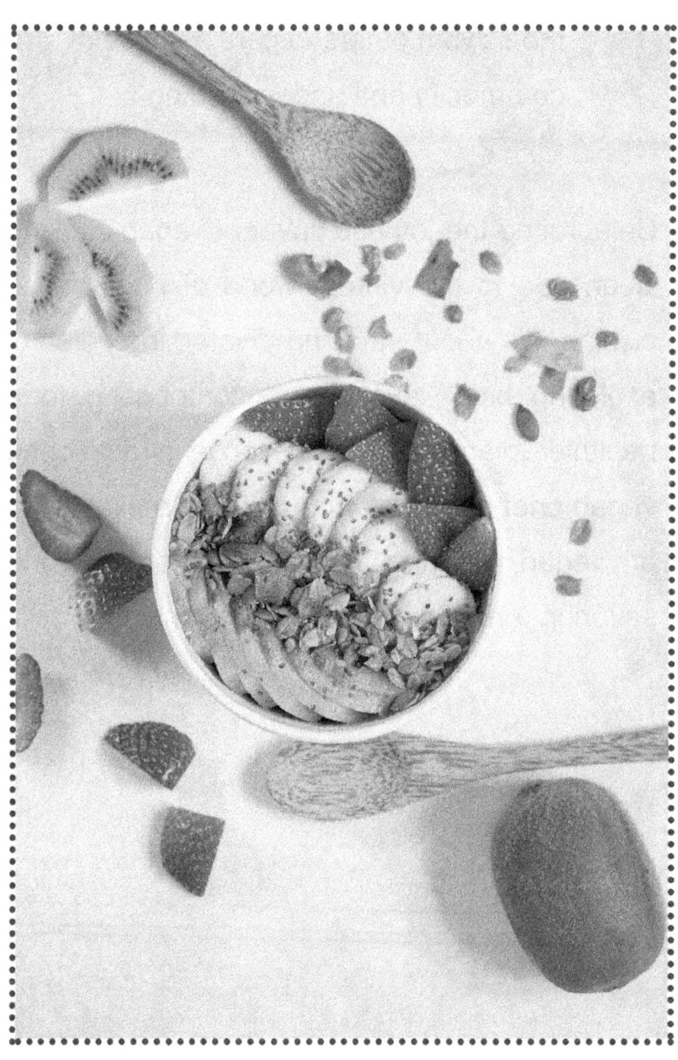

CONCLUSION

In the "Plant-Powered Kitchen Cookbook," readers embark on a flavorful and nutritious journey into the world of plant-based cuisine. This culinary masterpiece combines the art of cooking with the science of nutrition, offering a diverse range of recipes that celebrate the beauty and abundance of plant foods.

Throughout the cookbook, readers are guided through a holistic approach to cooking and eating, emphasizing the positive impact of a plant-based diet on health, the environment, and animal welfare. With its beautifully crafted recipes and insightful tips, this cookbook not only inspires seasoned vegans but also welcomes newcomers to the world of plant-based eating.

In conclusion, "Plant-Powered Kitchen Cookbook" is a culinary treasure trove that celebrates the joy of plant-based cooking while emphasizing its numerous benefits. Whether you're an experienced plant-based enthusiast or just beginning your journey, this cookbook is an invaluable resource for discovering the delicious world of plant-powered cuisine. With its tantalizing recipes and wealth of information, it's a must-have addition to any kitchen, guiding readers toward a healthier, more compassionate, and sustainable way .